Medicinal & Nutritional Supplement Healing

A guide for decision making.

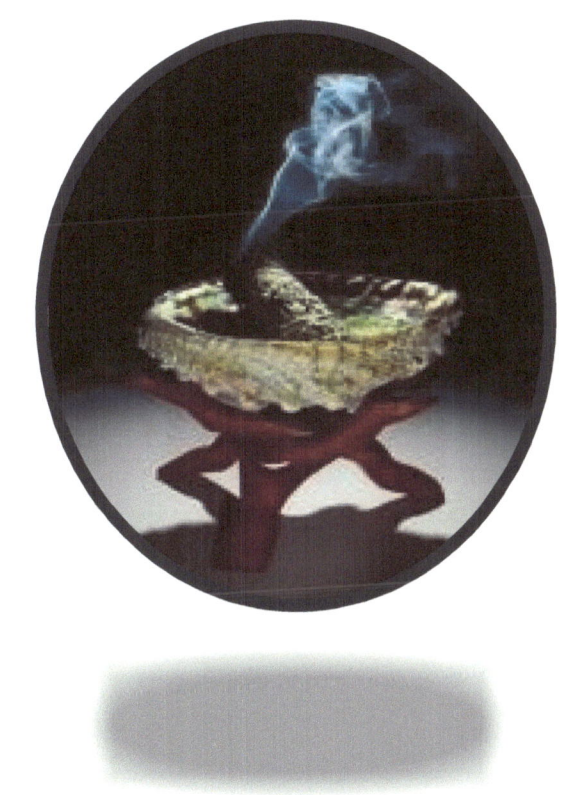

Mechell Turner, M.Ed. CCH CCE

July 2014

Introduction

Herbs, supplements, healing modalities all come in different forms and varieties. You and your health care provider should you help you chose which is the best way of supplementation and what forms to take or use. However, many people and even some health care providers, are confused on what each form is and they perform in and with the body. Also some herbs are used in different types of healing practices. This "Quick Guide" may help you decide what is best for you and your family. Any brands or pictures shown are not recommendations or endorsement of products or brands, just photos of what can be found in the market place. I have absolutely NO Financial interest in any of the companies, sources or brands shown here. I do, however, run my own herb and whole foods store in Peachland, NC. I do sell and make many supplements, just not all types.

Hopefully after reading these "briefs", you can understand the terminology used in the healing modalities and   our health care providers, and family.

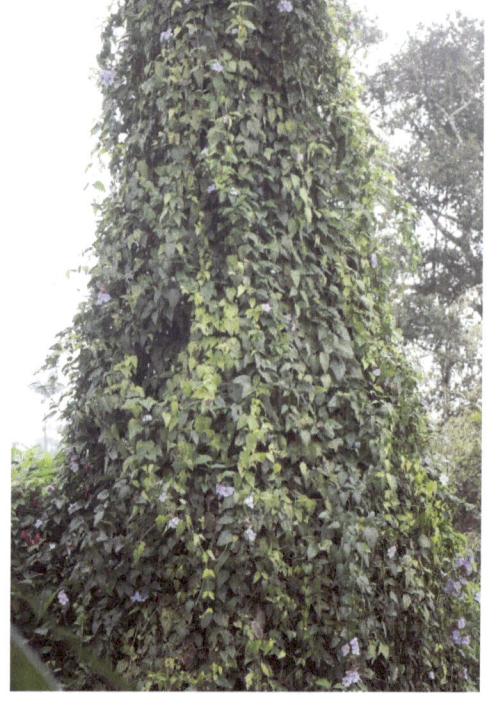

WARNING   WARNING   WARNING

ALLERGIC REACTIONS: DON'T WAIT
SEEK IMMEDIATE MEDICAL
ATTENTION. !!!!!!!!!!!!!!!!!

Discontinue use of any product,
Bag it up and take it with you to the
local emergency room, or urgent
care.

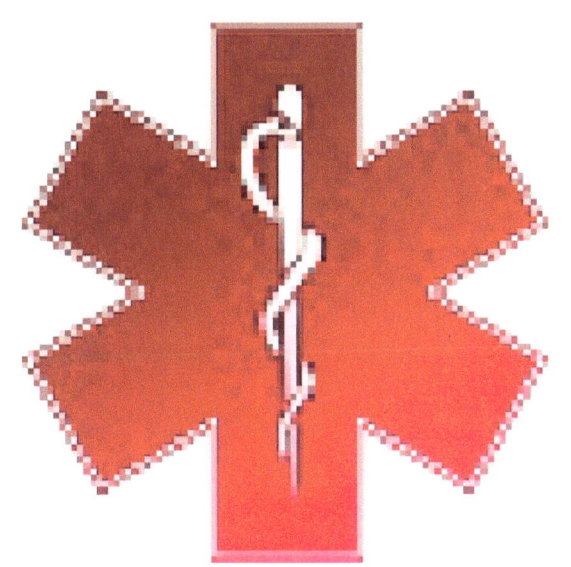

If your experience ITCHING, HIVES, WHEALTS, DIFFICUTLTY BREATHING,
SWELLING OF THE TONGUE OR THROAT, DIFFICULTY SPEAKING OR
CHANGES IN SKIN COLOR!!!!!!! THESE ARE SIGNS OF NEEDING HELP.
DIAL 911 OR YOUR LOCAL Emergency number.

**You can have an allergic reaction to any medication,
treatment or supplement, foods even if you have used them
before.**

Again seek medical Attention and do not try to self- treat.

Food First and best source of Health and Healing.

Foods are the first, easiest form of supplementation and nutrition.

Benefits and Basics:

1. **Human breast milk** is the ideal first food for all humans. Human milk is species specific for human babies. It is best and recommended for the first year or two of life. It has documented evidence of prevention of certain illnesses and provided immunities to the child. If not your own, donor human milk from a human milk bank or another mother, or an artificial baby milk (formula) should be used. (The rest is for another book.)
2. **Foods and meal** times can be enjoyable and enjoyed by all.
3. Provides the majority of nutrients, including trace elements for health and well-being.
4. **Best when** fresh as close to nature as possible, organic and local grown, fresh, home frozen, canned, then store purchased, are the ways you should shop. Meats, should be organic, homegrown without antibiotics, or hormones. Try raising something yourself if it be a few kitchen herbs and or a tomato plant. Getting into the food makes you healthier and eases the mind.
5. **Fats and oils** are not always the enemy, but amino acids are needed to build a human body, consume in moderation.

Methods: Raw, juiced, soups, steamed, baked, boiled, broiled, grilled or fried.

Drawbacks:

1. To get certain elements of some foods you have to eat huge amounts.
2. Large amounts of some foods can cause digestive upsets, including gas, heartburn, diarrhea or constipation.

3. You may tend to over eat and get unwanted calories.
4. Some foods are not recommended with certain medications. Ask your health care provider.
5. Moderation and well balanced variety diet is the key to health, and exercise to wellness and happiness.

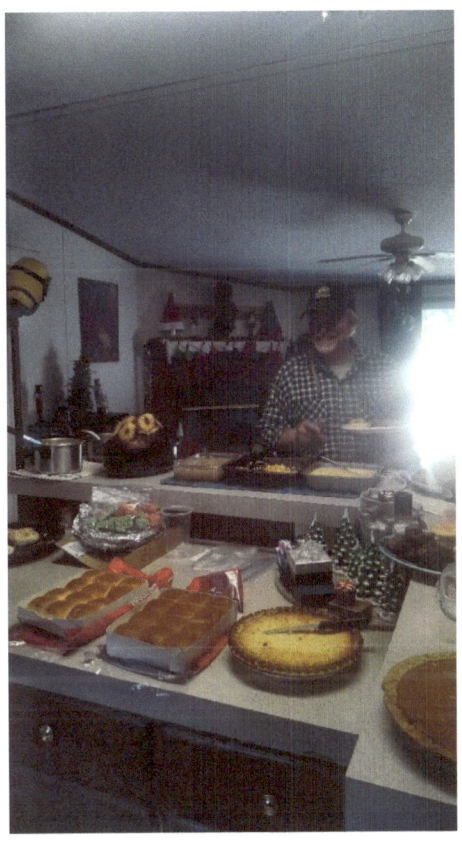

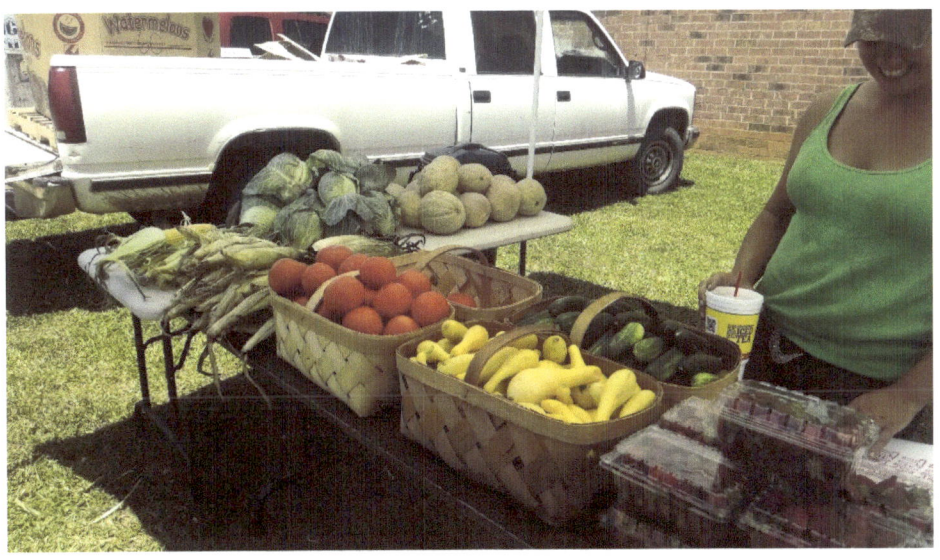

HERBAL TABLETS AND CAPSULES

Basics/Benefits

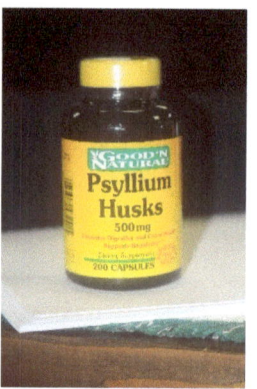

1. Come in many sizes and can vary from brand to brand.
2. Can be standardized to dosage and size.
3. Some powdered herbs/supplements can be capsuled at home. (It's a bit tricky and time consuming, but for some worth the effort.)
4. Some capsules can be broken open and used as tea.
5. May or may not come in child size dosages.
6. Decide if you want a single herb or combination/blend of herbs for your situation.

They come in these forms:

V-vegetarian,

VV vegan Vegetarian,

Capsules (gelatin), gel capsules are liquid/ oil filled

Hard Tablet, Chewable forms, Sub- lingual (under the tongue) forms.

Check labels for: expiration date, number of capsules or tablets, Number of capsules per dose, tablet/ capsule size, (U) Kosher, (P) parve, (Halal). Also check for additives and Certifications.

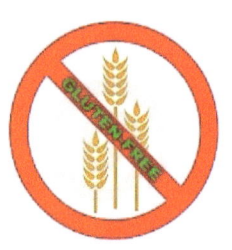
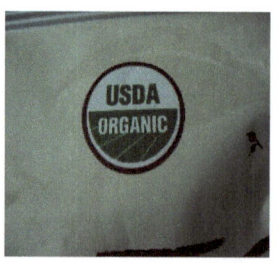
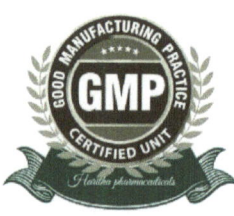
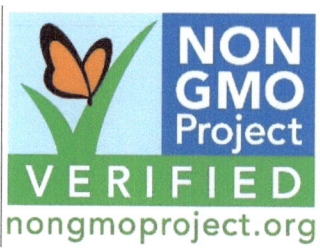

Tablets, capsules cont.

Particular Drawbacks:

1. **Check for** herb/ supplement and drug interactions.
2. **Check for fillers** they may contain, soy, dairy, gluten, wheat, eggs or nuts which can cause an allergic reaction.
3. **May be an** herbal or supplement blend. Know what you need or want. It is best to go with a good quality brand.
4. **Check for** any adulterations, or broken packaging.
5. **Must go through the digestive system.** You may think it is not working because you feel no immediate effect or reached the therapeutic dose. It takes time to break down substances to be absorbed in the intestine.
6. **May cause unwanted side effects:** gas, bloating, diarrhea, nausea or have a bitter aftertaste.
7. **Gel Capsules, tablets may** be hard to cut in half, you may lose some of the medicine. It may be a difficult size for swallowing.

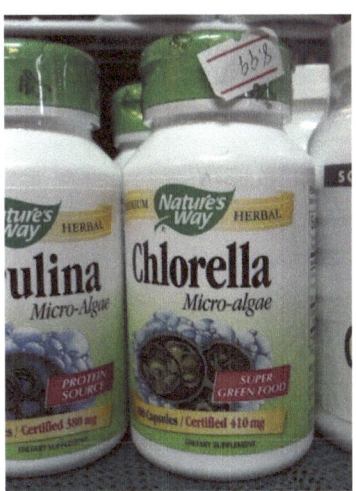

Herbal Teas

Basics and Benefits:

Herbal teas are the most basic of medicines and have been around since the dawn of time. It is basically the Plant/herb leaf, seed or root of a plant boiled or steeped in water.

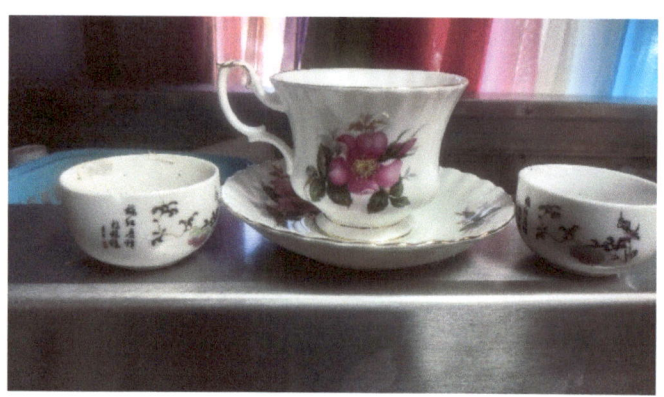

Can be made from all of or specific parts of the plant.

Tea is always **socially acceptable**

Medicinal beverage that is warming, hydrating and easy to administer.

True Tea is the leaf that is dried, fermented and cut from the Camilla Sinencis leaf. Rooibos and even coffee are teas.

Tisane- is a very weak non-caffeinated tea. Usually from the leaf of a plant. Its dilution alone differentiates it from a true tea, but is still of medicinal and hydrating. Some tisanes are or were used topically to treat wounds and sores.

Decoction- is the "mashing" of plant material first (usually using a mortar and pestle); then the plant is allowed to low boil for a long time to extract medicinal compounds, volatile oils, and scents. It's very strong and can be diluted to make tisanes or kept strong for teas and tincture making.

Infusion- is the extraction of the chemical properties with water, oil or alcohol by steeping. Most tea type infusions are a bit weaker than a decoction. However, oil and alcohol infusions usually take weeks but are strong. These types of infusions are great for making salves, balms and lotions.

Percolation- Is passing hot water over and through the plant material.

Fomentation/Plaster/Pilaster- Is made from the wet plant material mashed or crushed and blended. The material is then placed over the body, wound or affected area, with or without a cloth cover. Most plasters are covered to hold plant material in place.

Drawbacks, may include issues with tastes, texture, smell and oils forming on top of the water.

Fresh Plants – should be dry and dirt free to prevent contamination. They should also be correctly identified.

Dosage of compounds is difficult to calculate.

Some herbs, roots, leaves, and flowers do not give off all their medical compounds and properties well in water.

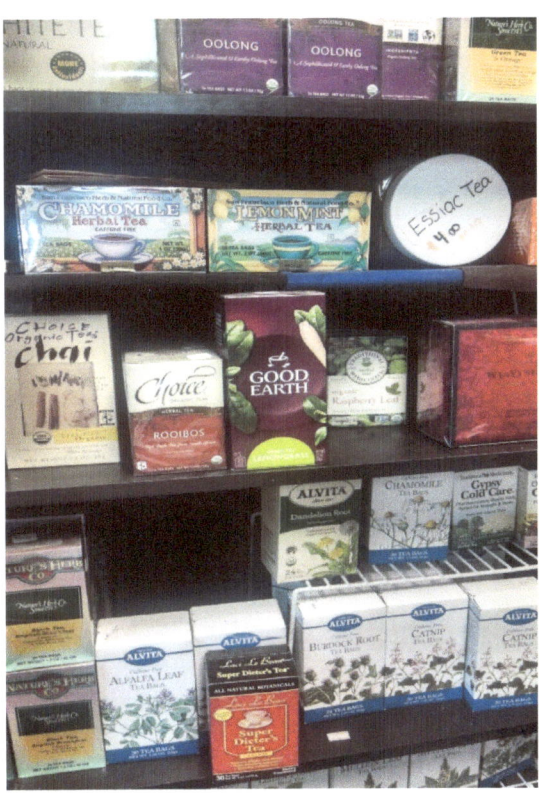

Herbal Tinctures/ Liquid Extracts

Basics: Tinctures or liquid extracts are single or multiple herbs (or other things) that have been soaked in fluid (other than water) such as grain alcohol, glycerin, or vinegar for several weeks. The liquid is then strained from the plant material. The liquid is then bottled. Dark bottles are the usual containers as it preserves the extraction better. Tinctures are also made by strongly boiled herbs, cooled, strained and then enough grain alcohol is added to preserve the extract. Strictly speaking tinctures are made from herbs which have been in a jar with alcohol.

Forms: Alcohol based, usually done with grain alcohol such as vodka, moonshine, or Everclear®. These have the longest shelf life. Alcohol tinctures are easy to make at home.

Vinegar based extracts, are also easy to make and suitable for all people. These have the next longest shelf life. Like all vinegars they are not always pleasant smelling and can develop a mother.

Glycerin extracts, have a shorter shelf life. They also are sweeter tasting and easy to give to children.

Benefits:

1. They can be taken at any time without regard for food intake.
2. Used sublingually (under the tongue) they are immediately absorbed into the bloodstream through the mucous membrane.
3. Easy to swallow.
4. Some can be used topically
5. You can make your own
6. Tinctures can be made from Fresh or dried herbs.

7. Doses are given in drops or droppersful.
8. Can be easily given to children and infants. (Caution with the dose and some herbs are not suitable for children.)
9. Alcohol tinctures stored correctly (in dark bottles, out of direct sunlight, slightly cool) may have the same shelf life as a good bottle of wine += 10 years.

Drawbacks:

1. Alcohol based tinctures may not be suitable for recovering alcoholics. They can be put into boiling tea or water to dissipate the alcohol.
2. Glycerin based tinctures have natural sugars in them.
3. Glycerin/vinegar based tinctures have a shorter shelf life.
4. Tinctures come in singles and blends, know what you need and seek professional guidance.

DO NOT confuse; tinctures with infused oils, or essential oils.

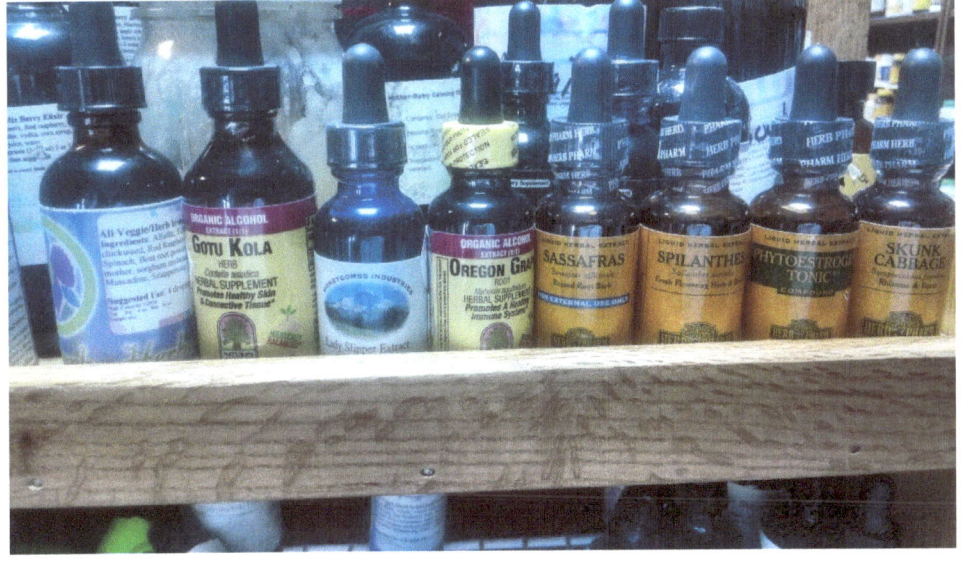

Homeopathy.

Definition:

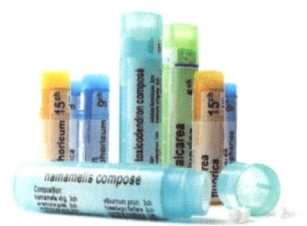

Homeopathy was described by 19th century Dr. Samuel Hahnemann where is used extreme dilutions of extracts of not only plants, but elements, animals and other things found in nature. Using the **Doctrine of Signatures,** of like cures like, he proposed that using minute amounts of a substance will cure the symptoms that a large amount of the same substance caused. His first was cinchona bark, which helped with malaria type symptoms. This is called a "proving." The remedy starts out with 1 part remedy to 10 parts menstruum. This is called a "mother tincture." This mother tincture is then diluted further with a single part of the mother tincture to (1 drop) to 99 parts of the menstruum, usually grain alcohol and then "succussed" or shaken to bring out the medicinal portion and energy of the tincture or plant. What is described is 1c. After enough succussions, the remedy is placed on the outside of a tablet, made of lactose. Each remedy deals with specific symptoms, a patient's personal constitution as well as the symptoms of the patient. Homeopathy is an energetic and vibrational system of medicine. It uses some herbs, but it also uses other things for healing, but it is NOT technically herbalism or herbal. Remedies can be found all over the world, and in some places it is a first go to rather than prescription medications.

Forms: generally pills, or little round pellets. You can buy homeopathic remedies in gel, liquid, forms as well.

Basics/ Benefits:

Generally regarded as safe, this includes, pets, infants, children, and some even with pregnancy and Breastfeeding/ Lactation.

Do not touch the outside of the pellets as the remedy is on the outside of the tablet. Pour into lid and then put under tongue.

Easy sublingual dosing. Remedies get into the bloodstream quickly via the mucous membrane.

Dilutions, are known as **potencies.** Which describe the number of dilutions, 10X 100's C1000's M, 10k MM. The higher the dilution the stronger the medicine.

Stored correctly the remedies can last for years. Dark bottles, or plastic, no extremes of temperatures. Never store remedies in the refrigerator.

Remedies always come in the Latin Binomial name. This insures that remedies are standard, reduces confusion and can be found from one country to another. ie. *Carbo Vegetabalis 6x, charcoal or coffea Cruda 30C is coffee*

Tissue salts: are the natural minerals and electrolytes that are found in the body.

Choosing the correct remedy is done two ways, by the individual's constitution, this is their overall body, emotions, and health. Your constitutional remedy is best found with the help of a professional homeopath.

Second is finding the remedy for the acute symptoms that the client is having. Say a right sided headache with sensitivity to noise. Or anxiety over a school test a student is about to undertake.

BACH FLOWER REMEDIES

These remedies are a homeopathic form of specific flowers and their essential oils to share their vibrational, emotional and physical healing properties of the plants themselves, rather than the individual patient's symptoms. These are used and dosed in Drops. Bach flower remedies are the most well-known brand of these remedies. Nature's Sunshine ® and others carry similar items.

Benefits:

Remedies can be used topically and orally with any client. They are safe for both animals, children and infants.

Dosage is usually in drops. They rarely react with other medications as they are used infrequently.

Rescue Remedy® or 5-flower remedy is great and essential to have in any medicine bag, for emergencies. I keep one in my purse and one in my medicine pouch.

Drawbacks:

If you are allergic to the specific flower/plant there is a rare possibility of allergic reaction. Since these are homeopathic doses it is uncommon.

Do not store in a hot car! The rubber tips can melt or dry out easily and heat can destroy the medicinal properties. In my healthcare practice, travelling with one is essential.

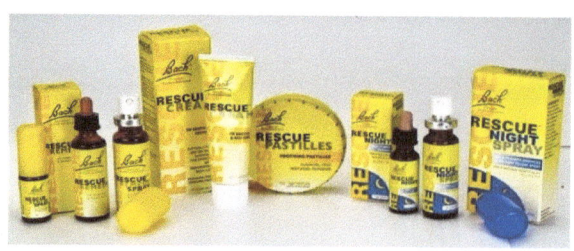

Essential Oils and Aromatherapy

Basics: Essential oils work through the limbic system in the brain. Science has shown that smell can trigger memories cognizant and healing functions. Oils are used in the treatment of illness, massage therapy, and inserted into soaps. Lotions, perfumes. And other oils. As you are reading this, think of some pleasant and unpleasant smells, skunk, coffee, roses, wet dog and see if you can find what they do.

Most essential oils are distilled from the plant or flower and are more the consistency of water or an extremely light oil. They are not thick and greasy. It takes about a 1000 pounds of rose petals to get an ounce of essential oil.

Some essential oils are pressed from the plant. But very few are.

Essential oils are not generally for human oral consumption. Even if they are orally consumed it is only in drops to several ounces of water. Only do so with the guidance of a health professional not just a sales person.

Look for bottles that have "therapeutic grade" on them.

Gas Chromatography is the standard test of excellence as each oil and plant has its own weight and smell.

Fragrance oils are NOT essential oils. These can be artificially made in a lab setting, they may or may not include the real oil. These can also be made with other oils and a little of the essential oil. Most of these are quite heavy and more "oily" than essential oils. These are the most likely to contain adulterants.

Infused oils are NOT essential oils. Infused oils are made from carrier oils, such as almond, jojoba, shea, olive or coconut oils. These oils have been place in a jar with raw or dried plant material, to infuse for several weeks to extract the healing properties from the herb as well as scent and taste. They can last quite a while and are used in salves lotions and creams, to where other essential oils and ingredients can be added. These are generally for used for eating as well as healing balms. Actually these are easy to make.

Many essential oils are quite **expensive** and they are used in drops in a carrier oil.

Carrier oil is another type of plant derived oil that is usually for eating or cooking, or other skin care. Examples are coconut, jojoba, almond, shea, olive, avocado, grapeseed oils. When using essential oils, they are usually put in these and go further.

Applying "Neat" is application of the oil alone. There are not many you really want to do this way because of cost and some oils can burn the skin. Lavender and tea tree are two oils that can be applied neat.

Best stored in Dark bottles, away from extreme heat and light. **Never** store in refrigerator.

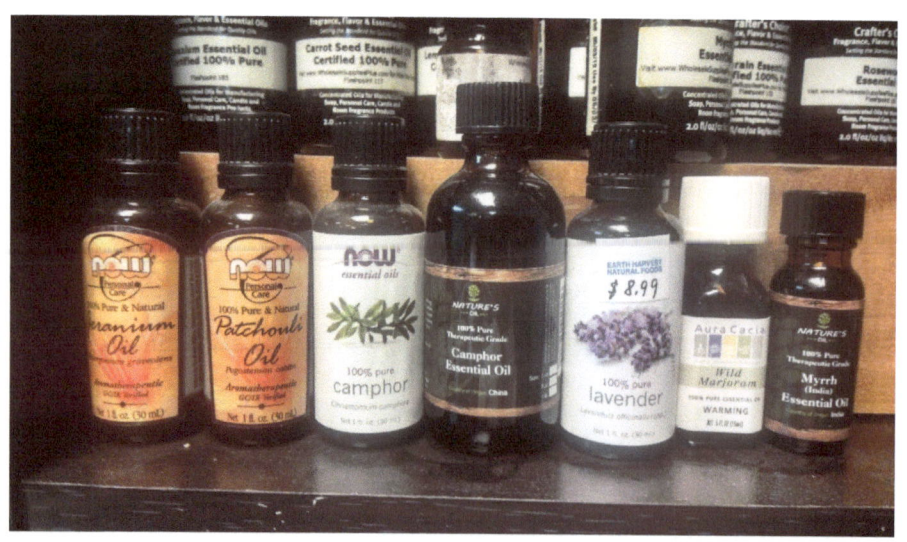

Traditional Chinese Medicine

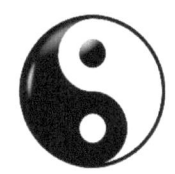

TCM is a system of medicine that is 3000+ years old. It uses foods, herbs, energetics and mind/body/spiritual relationships noted as "chi/qi to help one heal the body. Chi circulates in the body and is guided, healed and through specific meridians of the body. Imagine the points of the magnetism in the body lining up in a Magnetic Resonance imaging machine. These body issues are an imbalance of Yin/ yang, hot/cold and male/female. The body is governed by the 5 elements of nature: these are wood, earth, fire, water and metal. Each of these elements represent the various organs of the bod as well as its seasons, tastes and emotions. Healing and health are these elements and ones Chi being put into balance. TCM is most noted for using acupuncture/ acupressure, cupping, massage as well as foods, herbs, animal parts. If you are afraid of needles, many practitioners use a laser acupuncture machine with excellent results. In itself it not really painful. TCM is not considered extremely vegan since animal parts can and are used. These doctors, practioners also perform a myriad of tests, of pulse, tongue, and other body readings.

These practioners go through several years of study, medical school and pass a rigorous board exam to practice. You will find western doctors, chiropractors and others who are practicing acupuncture.

There are many Chinese formulas, singles that have proven themselves over the millennia. Many of these formulas come as teas, powders to decoct or as capsules that act synergistically with the mind, spirit, body healing mechanism. Many of the herbs carry their Latin binomial and English names.

EX. Fo-Ti= he shu wu = polygonum multiflorum

TCM continued.

Safety

With the correct practioner and study, acupuncture can be done safely on children, animals and pregnant women. It has been used in labor to eliviate pain and discomfort. It is also used to assist with turning babies in utero.

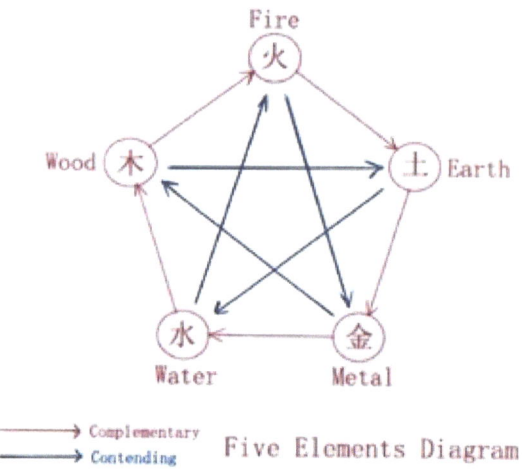

Five Elements Diagram

5 elements chart, acupuncture points model and sprained ankle with needles.

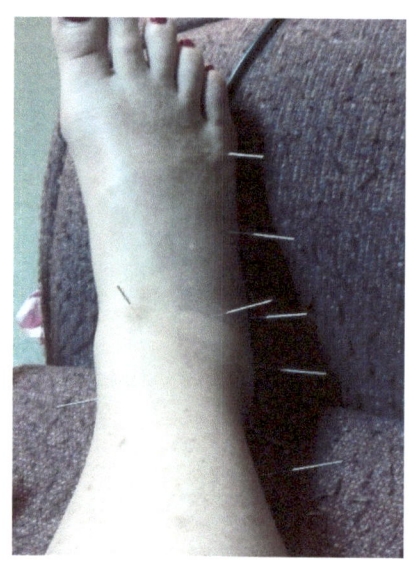

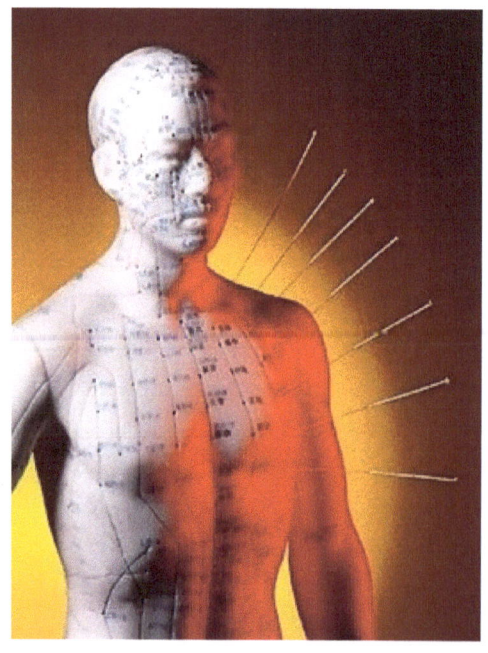

Ayurveda—"Life Knowledge"

Ayurveda is an East Indian form of medicine that works on diet along with the physical and spiritual constitution of the individual client. It is a 5000 year old system with its roots in the Hindu books of the Vedas: Rig Veda, Soma Veda, Yajur Veda and Hatharva Veda. They come together to form Ayurveda. The Vedas are revealed in a "constitutional assessment" of the individual. It not just the physical body (symptoms and appearance) but that of mind/ body/ spirit as they come to form a whole human being.

There are 3 primal forces of human wellness which are: Prana (breath), Agni (spirit) and Soma (Harmony). These also include the **5 elements of** matter which are earth, fire, water, air and ether (space).

This form of medicine seeks to describe the individuals using the three **Doshas (personality types/ humors)**. These humors are named Pitta, Kapha and Veda doshas. Each Dosha having its own set of parameters. Individuals are a combination of the three, but one in particular will stand out more than others.

To harmonize the doshas, one must harmonize the **7 Chakras** of the body. A chakra is an energy center of the body; these chakras also represent the body organs and systems. All energy and chakras in balance or harmony one can maintain long term healing, health and wellness.

The practice's philosophy and fundamental principle states that there is a Divine Life Force and Creative intelligence. This Light/life is eternal and constantly changes, but never dies. The individual should be able to use this essential life force or essential nature to find their purpose in life.

Most practitioners of the science of Ayurveda, take years of study and in many countries must pass a rigorous board exam to practice.

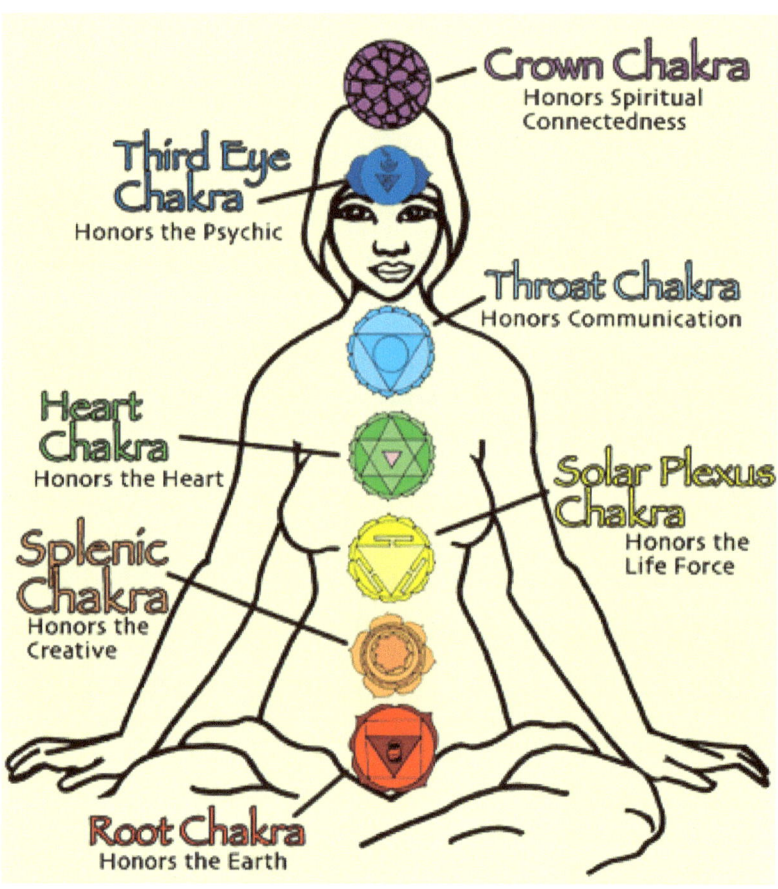

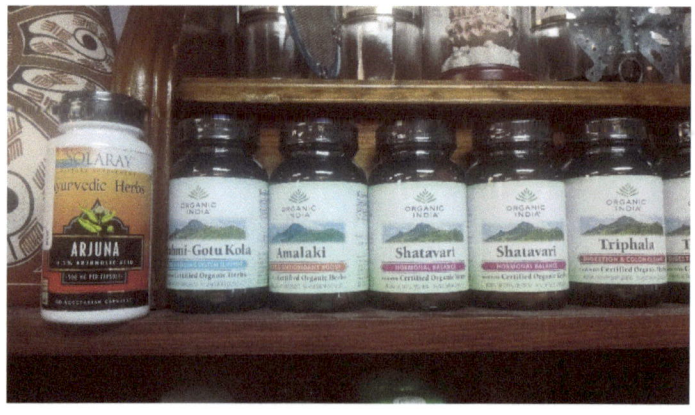

Native American – Indigenous Peoples' Medicine

Native American or Indigenous healing is not one particular style of healing per se. Most believe in the power of the spirit and balance of mind, body and soul. There is a divine life force who is eternal and is called the Creator, Great Mystery, etc. It is a set of beliefs and customs that are different by each tribe, clan or group. Healers, can be both spiritual healers and or physical healers.

Healers and others believe in a balance of all things in nature and in the body. We are all interconnected and to be respectful of Mother Earth, Father Sky and those who live upon the earth. Healers will bring their knowledge of plants, prayers, song and dance into the healing circle. Native medicine can be as simple as a prayer and a cup of tea or cleansings, and as Inca and Aztec even perform brain surgery. Both life and death are sacred and to be respected. Most healers of any sort do not brag or mention much that they are healers as is s gift and a learned art and science.

Herbs and other things are used. Most healers take years to study and learn from the elders of plants, animals, their uses, secrets and what not to use. Plants are also used for food, healing and offerings to aid in prayers to give sweet smelling savor to the Creator. Some are under the impression that indigenous folks worship the plants and animals. They are not worshiped, but seen as gifts from the creator. We are to be good stewards of nature and the gifts she brings. We are to observe plants, animals and the world around us to teach us respect for each other and the strengths and gifts they give to the peoples and be thankful for that gift of knowledge.

Some things that are used:

Drum is the heart beat of mother earth to ground us fully to her as from mothers we come to the earth when we cross over- die. Music is the gift of life. Dance and singing is a way of giving praise and worship to the Creator of Life himself.

Smoke to wing the prayers to heaven. This is usually some herb, in many traditions it is ceremonial white sage.

Offerings of: tobacco, sage, sweet grass, cedar or others depending on culture and tradition. Medicine wheel, gives us the 4 directions to offer such prayers and petitions. Certain services may use corn, other plants or animals.

Water, the source of life, for washing, cleansing, and sweat lodges etc.

Herbs, plants, to heal wounds, disease and other spiritual needs

Respect, honor, wisdom and compassion for fellow creatures, and humans and your relationship to the creator is the upmost in any circle.

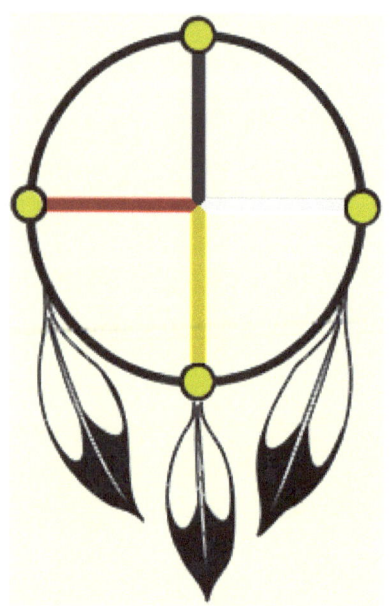
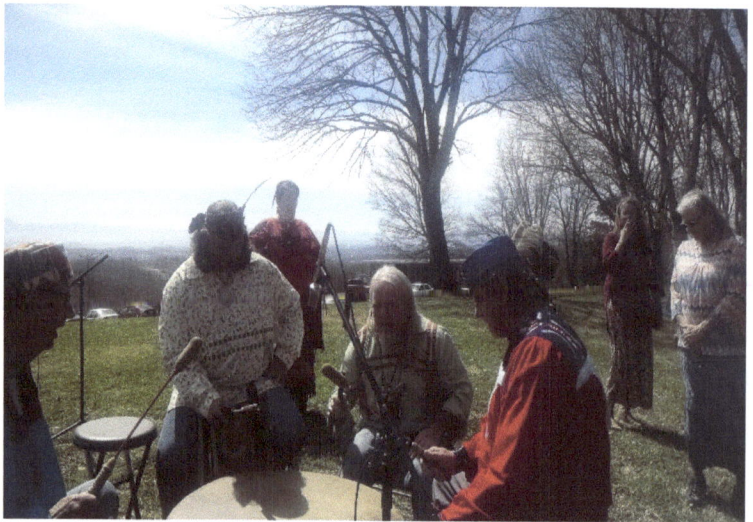

Free Trial: How to make your own.

Tincture and Infused Oil.

Tincture and infused oils take a similar process but different ingredients. Still you have to let them sit for about 6-8 weeks and shake every few days to "stir up the magic" so to speak.

For the Herbal tincture:

Gather a clean quart jar (glass works better) with a lid that will fit tight.

½ to one cup dried or fresh herb. If fresh make sure that it is clean dry and bug free.

2- 2 ½ cups 80 proof grain alcohol. For infused oil 2-2 ½ cups Olive oil.

For Fresh herbs: On sheet of wax paper or mortar and pestle grind and chop fresh herb to go into the clean dry jar.

Place herbs in the jar. And pour over alcohol until the jar is nearly full; leave about 1 inch of head (air) space. Shake well. Set aside in a cool dry and dark place (away from heat and light). On the 3rd day open and check and add a bit of alcohol (or oil) if needed, because the herbs soak it up. Put lid on tight. Shake once a week for 8 weeks. Use a strainer and coffee filter to strain off tincture in a larger jar or several smaller darker bottles and label. Return the grounds or left overs to the compost or ground.

Infused Oil. Gather the same stuff, except instead of alcohol a good quality olive, almond, jojoba or coconut oil. I personally do not use peanut oil due to allergies. Pour the oil over the herbs. Put on lid sake well and again, shake at least 1x a week. Do not store in refrigerator.

I hope you have enjoyed reading this small book. It is just meant to be a short quick reference guide to help you the consumer Decide what options for care are open to you and your families along with western medicine. There are great times for needs of a doctor, surgeon or experienced professional. But these healing modalities can aid in recovery, acute care and aid with needed lifestyle changes to make you healthier

Please check out my Website, WWW.NCsimplyherbal.net and like Simply Herbal on Facebook.

Mechell Turner, M.Ed. CCH, CCE, doula

Clinical Herbalist.

Owner, Simply Herbal

PO Box 479

Peachland, NC 28133